Yoga For Beginners: Learn the Right Poses For Peace

Become a Yoga Expert and Calm Your Mind

By: Rajesh Vishwani

9781632874481

I0413992

PUBLISHER'S NOTES

Disclaimer – Speedy Publishing, LLC

This publication is intended to provide helpful and informative material. It is not intended to diagnose, treat, cure, or prevent any health problem or condition, nor is intended to replace the advice of a physician. No action should be taken solely on the contents of this book. Always consult your physician or qualified healthcare professional on any matters regarding your health and before adopting any suggestions in this book or drawing inferences from it.

The author and publisher specifically disclaim all responsibility for any liability, loss or risk, personal or otherwise, which is incurred as a consequence, directly or indirectly, from the use or application of any contents of this book.

Any and all product names referenced within this book are the trademarks of their respective owners. None of these owners have sponsored, authorized, endorsed, or approved this book.

Always read all information provided by the manufacturers' product labels before using their products. The author and publisher are not responsible for claims made by manufacturers.

This book was originally printed before 2014. This is an adapted reprint by Speedy Publishing LLC with newly updated content designed to help readers with much more accurate and timely information and data.

Speedy Publishing, LLC©2014

40 E. Main Street #1156

Newark, Delaware

19711

Contact Us: 1-888-248-4521

Website: http://www.speedypublishing.com

REPRINTED Paperback Edition: ISBN: 9781632874481

Manufactured in the United States of America

DEDICATION

This book is dedicated to my father. Through his experiences, I realized that I was not fulfilling my purpose here on Earth. Through the practice of yoga I learned how to focus on the important things and to dispel the unnecessary clutter from my mind.

TABLE OF CONTENTS

Rajesh Vishwani

INTRODUCTION TO YOGA

As we march into this bright new millennium, we're constantly reminded of the fusion of east and west. Whether it's through satellite television programming that beams in productions from different cultures, enjoying books and music from distant lands that, only a generation or two ago, couldn't be accessed, and – of course – communicating with people across time and space through the Internet and other telecommunications advancements, the world has become a much smaller place. Indeed, when Marshall McLuan coined the term Global Village, even he probably didn't envision so much, so fast, so soon.

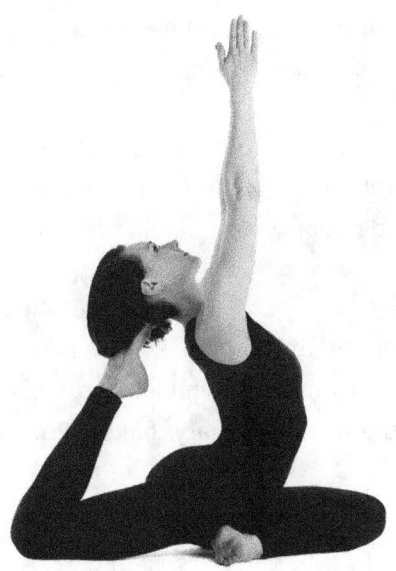

Riding the wave of information that now crisscross our tiny planet is something that has its roots in ancient history, yet is experiencing a blossoming in the west that continues to gain momentum with each passing year. Whether it's at a local YMCA or a lush spiritual retreat in the Everglades, Yoga is establishing itself as a mainstay in western culture; indeed, in the global culture.

However, many people are reluctant to experience the physical, emotional, and psychological health benefits of yoga; and there is really only one major reason for this: misinformation.

While many people might truly enjoy yoga and find it to be the side-effect free answer to a lot of their emotional and physical ailments, they just don't know enough about the subject to take that first step.

Furthermore, a stereotype out there that seems to persist despite evidence to the contrary is that yoga is a religious following; and that to experience its many health benefits somehow obliges one to renounce their faith or, worse, run away to some commune and eat tofu in between chanting sessions.

Well, yes, if you'd like to go to a retreat and enjoy tofu and chanting, that's probably possible (almost anything is possible, as long as it's legal and people want to do it, right?).

Yet that vision of yoga – people with shaved heads and handing flowers to strangers at the airport – is by no means the overall picture. Yoga is really a very simple, accessible, and in many countries around the world, ordinary thing to do.

In that light, this book is created with one goal in mind: to demystify yoga for you, and provide you with a clear, simple, and fun introduction to the topic.

If you've never been exposed to any kind of yoga (except for what you might have seen on television), then this book is for you!

Rajesh Vishwani

In addition, even if you have experienced some kinds of yoga (perhaps a friend dragged you to a class at the local recreation center all those years ago), this book will reignite your interest in the topic and reattach you into a mode of body movement and mind focus that has lived in ancient lands for millennium.

As you read through these sections, please bear in mind that there is absolutely no attempt here, directly or indirectly (or in any other way possible!) to endorse or promote any religious view. This is because the view of this book is the same view that is held by the world's foremost authorities on yoga: that it is not a religion. It does not have a dogma.

While there are indeed different schools and streams of yoga – there are actually thousands of them – they have all managed to coexist quite peacefully because, for the most part, yoga is not evangelical, which simply means that it does not seek to spread itself as part of its mission.

Please note that the statement above in no way criticizes or comments on evangelical orders, such as Evangelical Christianity; the point here is simply that the overwhelming majority of yoga movements does not consider spreading yoga to be a tenet of its identity.

Yet, while the yoga that is described in this book (and experienced in most of the world) is not a religion, it does very seamlessly fit into many people's existing religious framework.

In other words, if you are a Catholic, a Protestant, a Muslim, a Jew, a Sikh, or anything else and identify yourself as being a part of any faith at all, yoga doesn't ask you to replace that faith with someone else, or offer you a competing or contradictory view of what you already believe.

So please remember: yoga, as it is discussed and promoted in this book (and in virtually every book worth reading!) is not a religion.

As we'll begin to understand in the next section of this book, yoga is really nothing more, and nothing less, than harassing the power of human attention, and using it to benefit the body and mind. It is an approach to life, here and now.

CHAPTER 1- YOGA- WHAT IS IT?

What was I looking for that night in Bombay? The same thing I had been looking for as long as I can remember. The same thing all of us seek in one way or another. The "answer" to life, whatever that might mean. The "truth." The reason for living, dying, or being "here"at all."

- Beryl Bender Birch

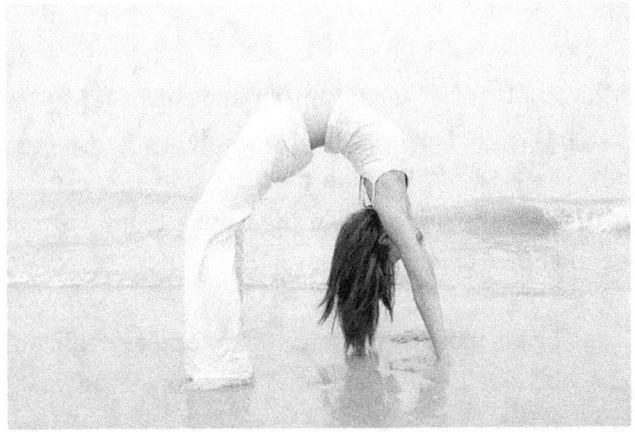

Yoga can seem like a complicated concept; or, at the very least, a dizzying array of physical manipulations that turn seemingly happy-looking human beings into happy looking human pretzels.

Or even more disconcerting, as we have alluded to in the Introduction, a stereotype does exist in places where the term yoga is synonymous with the cult, or some kind of archaic spiritual belief that compels one to quit their job, sell their house, and go live in the middle of nowhere.

In actual fact, Yoga is a very basic thing; and if you've had the opportunity to visit a country where it has been established for generations – India, Japan, China, and others – it's really rather, well, ordinary.

The practice of yoga came to the west back in 1893 when one of India's celebrated gurus, Swami Vivekananda, was welcomed at the World Fair in Chicago. He is now known for having sparked the West's interest in yoga.

Literally, the word yoga comes from the Sanskrit term Yug, which means: "to yoke, bind, join, or direct one's attention". At the same time, yoga can also imply concepts such as fusion, union, and discipline.

The sacred scriptures of Hinduism (an ancient belief system from India that has a global presence) also define yoga as "unitive discipline"; the kind of discipline that, according to experts Georg Feuerstein and Stephan Bodian in their book Living Yoga, leads to the inner and outer union, harmony and joy.

In essence, yoga is most commonly understood as conscious living; of tapping into one's inner potential for happiness (what Sankrit refers to as ananda).

What Yoga Isn't

Sometimes it's helpful to understand things by what they aren't; especially when dealing with a topic, like Yoga, that is quite easily misunderstood.

Authors and yoga scholars Feuerstein and Bodian help us understand yoga by telling us what it is NOT:

Yoga is NOT calisthenics (marked by the headstand, the lotus posture or some pretzel-like pose). While it is true that yoga involves many postures – especially in Hatha yoga – these are only intended to make people get in touch with their inner feelings.

Yoga is NOT a system of meditation – or a religion – the way many people are misled to believe. Meditation is only part of the whole process of bringing ourselves into the realm of the spiritual.

The Fundamental Nature of Yoga

Virtually all yogic science and philosophy states that a human being is but a fragment of an enormous universe, and when this human being learns to "communion" with this vastness, then he/she attains union with something that is bigger than him/her. This attachment or tapping into something bigger, thus enables one to walk the true path of happiness. By flowing along with the force, the individual is able to discover truth.

And with truth comes realization; but to attain realization, our words, thoughts and deeds must be based on truth. People attend courses on yoga and go to studios to learn new techniques in yoga, but yoga teacher Tim Miller said that "true yoga begins when [you] leave the studio; it's all about being awake and being mindful of your actions".

How Yoga affects Physical Health

Yoga does not see a distinction between the body and the mind; and this is an understanding that western psychology has also concluded for many years now (the link between mental health and physical health, and vice versa).

If you've come to this book looking to understand yoga as a means to help your body heal or improve, then please don't worry; you've come to the right place!

Yoga For Beginners
Yoga is indeed a process that involves releasing blocked tension and energy in the body, and helping make the muscles, tendons, joints, ligaments, and all other components work to their utmost potential.

Yoga believes that human beings are optimally designed, by nature, to be flexible and agile; and stiffness and lack of mobility only arrive when the body is unhealthy or out of alignment.

Therefore, countless people have found themselves in a yoga class, or on a yoga mat at home in front of a Yoga video or DVD, in the hopes of improving their physical health; and perhaps you may be one of them. If that's the case, then keep reading!

There are proven physical benefits of yoga, which include:

- Increased flexibility and range of motion

- Reduced pain in joints and muscles

- Stronger immune system

- Stronger lung capacity and therefore higher quality respiration

- Increased metabolism (which can lead to weight loss!)

- Higher quality of sleep (especially due to improved breathing and a more oxygenated body)

Given that certain yoga practices require postures to be mastered, yoga has always helped promote the body's flexibility; it also helps in lubricating the joints, ligaments and tendons. Yoga detoxifies by increasing the flow of blood to various parts of the body. It helps tone and invigorates muscles that have grown flaccid and weak.

Rajesh Vishwani

So please do keep in mind that, while yoga is often discussed in terms of its mental approach, there are clear and proven physical benefits that are a part of this approach.

Therefore, if weight loss is your goal, or the ability to shovel the snow in winter without having your back ache for days, then yoga is as viable an option to you as it is for the stressed-out corporate executive who needs to find a strategy for coping with the craziness if her busy life!

"Yoga is thus not just twisting the body to perform certain asanas or postures, but balancing the mind and body, making it more receptive to the universal life force pouring from the Supreme Self. Hence, be truthful, do your duty and love all, along with a few asanas daily to keep yourself on the path of evolution."

CHAPTER 2- IS YOGA BENEFICIAL?

As we've repeatedly pointed out in this book (and probably started to bore you with; sorry!), yoga is not a religion. It can be religious if one wants it to be, and it can co-exist with an existing religious belief. But yoga itself is not religious in the sense that it focuses on belief or faith.

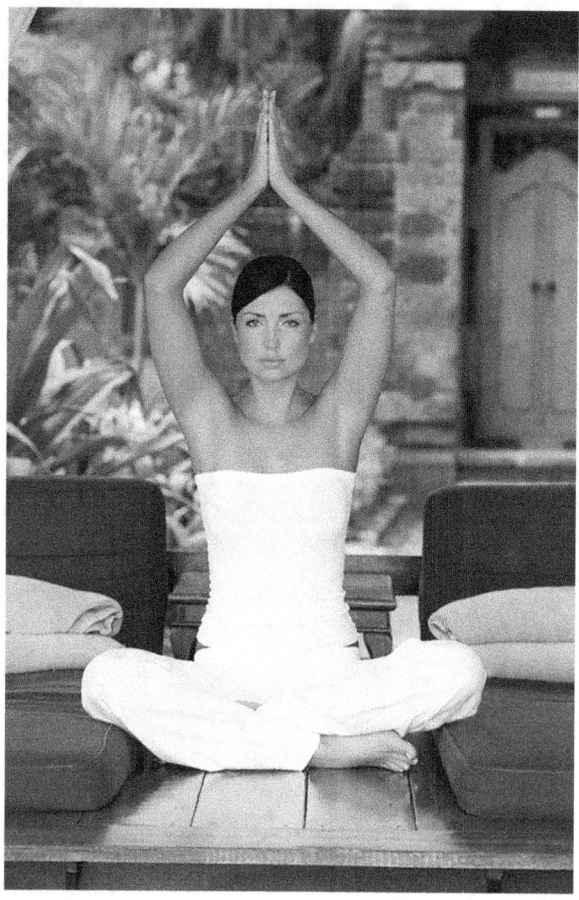

Yoga is a science; and indeed, in many places in the world (such as India), it is referred to as a science. This is not mere playing with words; it truly is approached as a science, which means that it is understood in terms of the scientific method.

Yogic science seeks to verify cause and effect, and build principles based upon objective observations. Indeed, in many places in the world, to be a yogi master of any credibility, one must be highly educated in the sciences, including physics and the biological sciences.

This discussion on yoga as science is important for us to have here, because it allows us to sensibly ask the question: what are the benefits of yoga? After all, if yoga is a faith or a belief, then asking this question isn't fair; because it's one that yoga cannot answer in terms that we can objectively understand.

Yet (again... sorry!) yoga is a science; as empirical and pragmatic as kinesiology, or exercise science, which seeks to understand how the body acts and reacts to changes in the internal physical environment. And even simpler than any of this: each of us has a right to ask the basic question why should I bother doing this yoga thing? Before we should be asked to consider experiencing it for ourselves.

Indeed, while the experience of yoga cannot be reduced to words – just as reading a book on preparing for a marathon isn't going to actually physically prepare you to run a marathon – the goals and principles of yoga can easily be discussed.

Benefits of Meditation (Mayo Clinic)

Meditation is used by people who are perfectly healthy as a means of stress reduction. But if you have a medical condition that's worsened by stress, you might find the practice valuable in reducing the stress-related effects of allergies, asthma, chronic pain and arthritis, among others.

Yoga For Beginners

Yoga involves a series of postures, during which you pay special attention to your breathing — exhaling during certain movements and inhaling with others. You can approach yoga as a way to promote physical flexibility, strength and endurance or as a way to enhance your spirituality.

Advantages of Practicing Yoga

Yoga through meditation works remarkably to achieve harmony and helps the mind work in synchronization with the body. How often do we find that we are unable to perform our activities properly and in a satisfying manner because of the confusions and conflicts in our mind weigh down heavily upon us?

Stress is the number one suspect affecting all parts of our physical, endocrinal and emotional system. And with the help of yoga this things can be corrected.

At the physical level, yoga and its cleansing practices have proven to be extremely effective for various disorders.

Listed below are just some of the benefits of yoga that you can get:

Yoga is known to increase flexibility; yoga has postures that trigger the different joints of the body. Including those joints that are not acted upon with regular exercise routines.

Yoga also increases the lubrication of joints, ligament and tendons. The well-researched yoga positions exercise the different tendons and ligaments of the body. It has also been found that the body which may have started doing yoga being a rigid one may experience a quite remarkable flexibility in the end on those parts of the body which have not been consciously worked upon.

Yoga also massages all organs of the body. Yoga is perhaps the only exercise that can work on through your internal organs in a thorough manner, including those that hardly get externally stimulated during our entire lifetime.

Yoga acts in a wholesome manner on the various body parts. This stimulation and massage of the organs in turn benefit us by keeping away disease and providing a forewarning at the first possible instance of a likely onset of disease or disorder. One of the far-reaching benefits of yoga is the uncanny sense of awareness that it develops in the practitioner of an impending health disorder or infection. This in turn enables the person to take pre-emptive corrective action

Yoga offers a complete detoxification of the body. It gently stretches the muscles and joints as we; as massaging the various organs, yoga ensures the optimum blood supply to various parts of the body. This helps in the flushing out of toxins from every nook and cranny of your body as well as providing nourishment up to the last point. This leads to benefits such as delayed ageing, energy and a remarkable zest for life.

Yoga is also an excellent way to tone your muscles. Muscles which have been flaccid and weak are stimulated repeatedly to shed excess fats and flaccidity.

But these enormous physical benefits are just a "side effect" of this powerful practice. What yoga does is harmonize the mind with the body and these results in real quantum benefits.

It is now an open secret that the will of the mind has enabled people to achieve extraordinary physical feats, which proves beyond doubt the mind and body connection.

In fact, yoga = meditation, because both work together in achieving the common goal of unity of mind, body and spirit which can lead to an experience of eternal bliss that you can only feel through yoga.

The meditative practices through yoga help in achieving an emotional balance through detachment.

This in turn creates a remarkable calmness and a positive outlook, which also has tremendous benefits on the physical health of the body.

The Connection between Mind and-Body

Yoga centers on the mind-body connection. This mind-body harmony is achieved through three things:

A. Postures (asanas)

B. Proper breathing (pranayama)

C. Meditation

Mind and body draw inspiration and guidance from the combined practices of asanas, breathing, and meditation. As people age (to yogis, ageing is an artificial condition), our bodies become susceptible to toxins and poisons (caused by poor environmental and dietary factors).

Yoga helps us through a cleaning process, turning our bodies into a well synchronized and well-oiled piece of machinery.

Physical Benefits of Yoga

By harmonizing these three principles, the benefits of yoga are attained. And just what are these benefits? These benefits include:

- Equilibrium in the body's central nervous system

- Decrease in pulse rate

- Respiratory and blood pressure rates

- Cardiovascular efficiency

- Gastrointestinal system stabilization

- Increased breath-holding time

- Improved dexterity skills.

- Improved balance

- Improved depth perception

- Improved memory

Yoga-Psychological Benefits

As noted above, Yoga also delivers an array of psychological benefits; and in fact, this is a very common reason why people begin practicing it in the first place. Perhaps the most frequently mentioned psychological benefit of yoga is an improved ability to manage stress. Yoga diminishes an individual's level of anxiety, depression, and lethargy; thus enabling him/her to focus on what spiritual and important: achieving balance and happiness.

Following a Healthy Lifestyle

There is some very interesting psychology behind this that students of western thinkers (e.g. Freud, Jung, Fromm, etc.) will find familiar and, indeed, quite rational.

Yoga For Beginners

When an individual decides to be happy, something within that person activates; a kind of will or awareness emerges. This awareness begins to observe the jungle of negative thoughts that are swimming constantly through the mind.

Rather than attacking each of these thoughts – because that would be an unending struggle! – Yoga simply advises the individual to watch that struggle; and through that watching, the stress will diminish (because it becomes exposed and thus unfed by the unconscious, unobserving mind!).

At the same time, as an individual begins to reduce their level of internal negativity, subsequent external negative behaviors begin to fall of their own accord; habits such as excessive drinking, emotional overeating, and engaging in behaviors that, ultimately, lead to unhappiness and suffering.

With this being said, it would be an overstatement to imply that practicing yoga is the easiest way to, say, quit smoking, or to start exercising regularly. If that were the case, yoga would be ideal! Yoga simply says that, based on rational and scientific cause and effect relationships that have been observed for centuries, that when a person begins to feel good inside, they naturally tend to behave in ways that enhance and promote this feeling of inner wellness.

As such, while smoking (for example) is an addiction and the body will react to the lessening of addictive ingredients such as tar and tobacco (just to name two of many!), yoga will help the process. It will help provide the individual with the strength and logic that they need in order to discover that smoking actually doesn't make them feel good.

Rajesh Vishwani

In fact, once they start observing how they feel, they'll notice without a doubt that instead of feeling good, smoking actually makes one feel quite bad inside; it's harder to breathe, for one.

Now, this book isn't an anti-smoking book, and if you've struggled with quitting smoking then please don't be offended by any of this; there is no attempt here at all to imply that quitting smoking is easy, or just a matter of willpower.

Scientists have proven that there is a true physical addiction that is in place, alongside an emotional addiction that can be just as strong; perhaps even stronger.

The point here is simply to help you understand that yoga can help a person make conscious living choices that promote healthy and happy living. This can include:

- Quitting smoking

- Reducing excess drinking

- Eating healthier

- Getting more sleep

- Reducing stress at work (and everywhere else for that matter)

- Promoting more harmonious relationships all around

Please remember: yoga doesn't promise anyone that these things will simply happen overnight. At most, yoga is the light that shows you how messy things in the basement really are; and once that light is on, it becomes much more straightforward – not to mention efficient and time effective – to clean things up!

Yoga- Emotional Benefits

Yoga has also been hailed for its special ability to help people eliminate feelings of hostility and inner resentment. As a result of eliminating these toxic emotions, the doorway to self acceptance and self actualization opens.

How Yoga Helps With Pain Management

Pain management is another benefit of yoga. Since pain and chronic pain are conditions that affect all of us at some point, understanding the positive link between yoga and pain management could be invaluable.

It can also be financially valuable, since the pain medication industry is a multi-billion dollar marketplace and many people, especially as they age, find that their insurance or government coverage won't cover some pharmaceutical and over-the-counter pain relief medications. The website www.lifepositive.com provides some illuminating information on yoga and pain management:

Yoga is believed to reduce pain by helping the brain's pain center regulate the gate-controlling mechanism located in the spinal cord and the secretion of natural painkillers in the body.

Breathing exercises used in yoga can also reduce pain. Because muscles tend to relax when you exhale, lengthening the time of exhalation can help produce relaxation and reduce tension.

Awareness of breathing helps to achieve calmer, slower respiration and aid in relaxation and pain management. Yoga's inclusion of relaxation techniques and meditation can also help reduce pain. Part of the effectiveness of yoga in reducing pain is due to its focus on self-awareness.

Rajesh Vishwani
This self-awareness can have a protective effect and allow for early preventive action.

CHAPTER 3- YOGA- THE VARIOUS TYPES

It's funny looking at it this way, but one of the things that has promoted the spread of yoga in the west, is the same thing that can sometimes prevent someone from truly exploring it and therefore experiencing its health benefits. This thing is the variety.

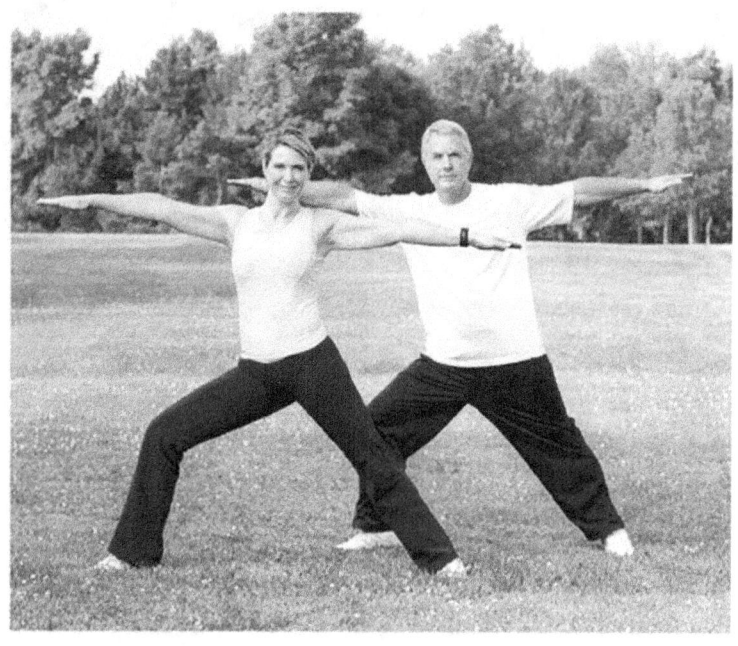

Sometimes when there is only one of something – such as one idea, or one language, or one anything – it's hard for that thing to spread outside of those who abide by it, agree with it, or simply want it to continue existing.

Yet when there are multiple ideas and concepts, the chances of it spreading increase; there are just more people out there who will be able to access it, talk about it, and indeed, make it a part of their life.

What does this have to do with yoga? Well, there are many different types of yoga; and the reason for this, as we initially discussed, is that yoga isn't a religion; it's an approach to being alive. As such, it's very agile and flexible (no pun intended!) and carries well across culture, country, and religious boundaries.

Thanks to its diversity and different facets and types, yoga has spread very swiftly through the western world over the last 110 years or so; and is spreading faster now than ever before (many western companies will now pay for yoga classes as part of an enhanced health benefits program).

Yet this very diversity has led to some confusion; and people who have been exposed to one kind of yoga might accidentally think that they've seen it all. This is more worrisome, of course, when one has been exposed to a kind of yoga that – for whatever reason – they did not like, or perhaps, weren't quite ready for (just as how some people might turn away from a fitness program if they aren't in the right frame of mind to see it through).

So if you've experienced yoga, or seen it on television, read about it in a newspaper, or overheard a friend or colleague talk about it, then please be aware that there's a very good chance that you haven't been exposed to all that there is (which is wonderful, because it means that this next section will be very interesting and informative for you!).

Yogic scholars Feuerstein and Bodian note seven major types of yoga. In no particular order, they are:

    I.   Hatha yoga

II. Raja yoga

III. Karma yoga

IV. Bhakti yoga

V. Jnana yoga

VI. Tantra yoga

Let's look at each one of these in turn.

Hatha Yoga

Graham Ledgerwood, who has been teaching yoga and mysticism for over 30 years, says that Hatha yoga is practiced in the west, mostly for health and vitality, and is the most popular in western society.

Ha is a Sanskrit term meaning sun, so Hatha yoga according to Ledgerwood is a "marvelous means of exercising, stretching, and freeing the body so it can be a healthy, long-lived, and vital instrument of the mind and soul".

Hatha yoga is known as the 5000 year old system which was used to increase the healthy body, mind and spirit. People who do Hatha Yoga combine the stretching exercises of the asanas into their practice. It includes the mental concentration and breathing techniques.

The Lotus position from Asanas is being used in practicing Hatha Yoga.

The goal of applying Hatha Yoga is just the same as using other kinds of Yoga. It aims to blend the human spirit with the peaceful spirit of the Universe. With this practice, the person doing the Yoga exercise increases their spiritual, mental, physical and emotional health and aspect.

Doing Hatha Yoga gives you peace and keeps your environment and the world as one. In doing yoga, including all types of yoga, concentration is the root or main ingredient for a successful yoga

All other types of Yoga have some similarities in one way or the other. The main focus of Hatha Yoga is to prepare the body to give in so that the spirit will be able to absorb and accomplish its mission. The spirit is responsible in lifting and enlightening. When the spirit is enlightened, the mind is relaxed and it throws away all stress and pain. The body does too.

Too many people get confused because they do not understand that if your body is not healthy and unfit; your spirit cannot successfully accomplish the task. So the goal of Hatha Yoga is perfect to apply if your spirit is weak.

Hatha Yoga will help encourage your body to move and advance positively to a level in which the spirit will be able to work properly. Your spirit and body needs to respond positively so that the mind will be able to keep up with a good concentration.

When people hear of the word Yoga, Hatha Yoga will come to their minds first. Hatha Yoga is popular and it is the popular branch of Yoga. In fact, the other style of yoga such as the Kundalini, Ashtanga, Bikram and Power Yoga has originated from Hatha Yoga.

Hatha Yoga is known as the vehicle for the soul. It is responsible for driving the body and the spirit in the universe. Just imagine soaring to the universe and feel no gravity at all. That is just so relaxing and tempting.

Concentration is something that is hard to maintain and recover. If you find yourself easily distracted by outside forces, Hatha Yoga might work to fight it.

The best thing about practicing Hatha Yoga is that it helps you find out for yourself that there is a divine light that shines in you. Not only does it enlighten you, but it can help you become stronger, relaxed and flexible.

The exercise involved in doing Hatha Yoga allows the spiritual energy to flow through the open energy channels. This will be possible if the mind, body and spirit are working well and has harmony. Of course, maintaining a healthy body is the most important of all. If your body is weak, your mind and spirit is affected too

When you practice Hatha Yoga, you can easily cope up with stress and relieve some pain and tension. Sometimes, work leaves you wasted and exhausted, so you need to relax once in a while. Hatha Yoga is the best remedy to release that pain and tension.

Perfecting the postures in Hatha yoga has two objectives:

Meditating

People need at least one posture that they can be totally comfortable with, for a long period of time. The more postures you can master, the better you are able to cultivate deeper meditation techniques.

Renewing body's energies for optimum health

Raja Yoga

Similar to classical yoga, Raja Yoga is considered the "royal path" to unifying the mind and body. Raja yoga is considered by some to be a rather difficult form of yoga, because it seeks enlightenment through direct control and mastery of the mind.

People who can concentrate well and enjoy meditation are best suited to Raja yoga. This type – or branch – of yoga has 8 limbs:

- Moral discipline

- Self-restraint

- Posture

- Breath control

- Sensory inhibition

- Concentration

- Meditation

- Ecstasy

Karma Yoga

Karma yoga involves selfless action. The word karma itself means action – all actions that come from the individual beginning from his birth until his death. Most importantly, karma is the path to doing the right thing. Hence the practice of karma yoga means giving up the ego to serve God and humanity.

Karma yoga comes from the teachings of the Bhagavad Vita, which is sometimes respectfully referred to as "the New Testament of Hinduism". Service to God through serving others is the foundation of Karma Yoga.

Bhakti Yoga

Sri Swami Sivananda says:

"Mark how love develops. First arises faith. Then follows attraction and after that adoration. Adoration leads to suppression of mundane desires. The result is single-mindedness and satisfaction. Then grow attachment and supreme love towards God.

In this type of highest Bhakti all attractions and attachment which one has for objects of enjoyment are transferred to the only dearest object, God. This leads the devotee to an eternal union with his Beloved and culminates in oneness."

Bhakti yoga is thus seen as divine love. As a force of attraction, Swami Nikhilananda and Sri Ramakrishna Math say that love operates on three levels:

- Material

- Human

- Spiritual

These two yogis further explain that love is a creative power, and this creative power pushes us to seek joy and immortality. In their own elegant and precise words:

Love based upon intellectual attraction is more impersonal and enduring... It is a matter of common observation that the more intellectually developed the life of a person is, the less he takes pleasure in the objects of the senses.

Jnana Yoga

Jnana yoga is the path to wisdom. Graham Ledgerwood defines Jnana as "emptying out" the mind and soul of delusions so that individuals can be attuned to reality, releasing all thoughts and emotions until the individual is transformed and enlightened.

Jnana yoga is one of the four main paths that lead directly to self-realization (philosophy of Advaita vedanda). By crushing the obstacles of ignorance, the student of Jnana yoga experiences God.

Concepts such as discernment and discrimination are highly regarded in Jnana yoga, where the student or a devotee identifies himself as separate from the components of his environment. "Neti-Neti" is also a principle inherent in Jnana Yoga. Literally, it means "not this, not this" and by removing objects around, what's left is just YOU and only you.

Tantra Yoga

A seventh type of yoga that many people have heard about, and indeed, is quite curious about, is tantra yoga.

Tantra yoga is considered by some to be most oriental of all yoga branches. It is often misunderstood as consisting exclusively of sexual rituals. It involves more than sex: it is the path of self-transcendence through ritual means, one of which is just consecrated sexuality. Some Tantric schools actually recommend a celibate lifestyle after a certain point.

Tantra literally means "expansion." A Tantra devotee expands all his levels of consciousness so he/she can reach out to the Supreme Reality. Tantra yoga aims to awaken the male and female aspects within a person to trigger a spiritual awakening.

Tantra yoga is more concentrated on the spiritual healing and most of all the integration of the body, mind, and spirit. In India, it is an ancient tradition that sexuality is an important and significant phase to be able to achieve a certain degree of enlightenment.

In Western religious norms, sexual pleasures and desires are not inclined or associated with spirituality. With these differences in traditions, there exists a fine line between their feelings and attitude towards sexuality along with spirituality.

However, in Eastern philosophy, they celebrate and rejoice in the splendor and glory of creation. And later on, they have developed a study or science for understanding how to get the most of this therapeutic and wonderful experience. Energy is known and considered to be the source of life in Tantra.

Furthermore, they consider the sexual energy and urge as great and sacred energy. There exists a few of the many exercises that help in the performance on the sexual aspect as well as some dietary adjustments. Some of these physical exercises include contractions, breathing and holding certain positions.

There are so many benefits that can be obtained by performing these various physical exercises. Some of these include improved prostate functioning and enhanced and improved sexual performance. Another benefit is improved sexual stamina when engaging in sexual intercourse.

There are also different kinds of exercises. Aside from the physical exercises, there are psycho-spiritual exercises. These exercises are ways to develop mediation on unconditional love and desire. As a result, this can make sexual activities less anxious and awkward, aside from that, the pressure to perform and move is minimized.

It is said that the most fascinating sexual experience is giving in completely to your partner or lover what he or she really wants.

Expectations may be high, so one must perform and must do something about it.

Through mediation and proper exercises, one can think of the various ways which he can satisfy his lover. When one is focused and concentrated on giving what your lover really wants is an experience which can strengthen your relationship with each other, moreover, you will receive the satisfaction you had always wanted. There are a few exercises which can help you a lot I focusing on your sexual performance.

By repeating some mantras and chants together with breathing exercises and proper meditation, one can achieve these benefits.

There are also numerous ways to take your foreplay to the highest level. With healing massages and gentle stroking, one can receive a rewarding experience that can stimulate both physical and spiritual and healing in different ways.

Reiki or energy channeling healing is practiced before engaging in a sexual activity. This is known to heighten the sexual pleasure in an intercourse. It is an Eastern healing art whereby one partner channels his energy to the other.

Through tactile stimulation, healing is achieved and both the physical and spiritual aspect is enhanced. In this manner, both of you can achieve a deeper state of relaxation and meditation which is very helpful to couples and partnerships.

Advice for Beginners

As you now know (if you didn't know it when you started reading, that is!), yoga is a very interesting and ancient approach of uniting the body and the mind. It has proven health benefits, including emotional and physical improvements.

The chances therefore are, if you're on the verge of starting a yoga program (perhaps at a local center or you've purchased a video or DVD and want to try it at home), you're excited, optimistic, and anxious to get going!

Yet it's wise to note that, before going into yoga practice, you should ask yourself some important questions. These questions don't have a right or wrong answer.

They are merely meant to stimulate your own thoughts and give you the mindset that you need in order to succeed as a student of yoga for the long term.

Here are the basic questions that you should ask before starting any yoga program:

- What are my reasons for starting a yoga program? Are they realistic?

- If my yoga program involves some degree of physical strain, such as certain postures in Hatha yoga, have I received medical clearance from a qualified and certified health professional to ensure that I don't injure myself?

- Are my goals for pursuing a yoga program (or programs) clear and positive? Do I know what I want to achieve?

- Am I prepared to commit the time necessary to really get the most of out of my yoga experience?

- Are there people around me who might negatively try and talk me out (or mock me out) of pursuing this path of personal development? Should I either avoid such people, or ask them to respect what I'm choosing to do?

Please note that these are just basic questions; and this isn't an exhaustive list. The point here is really that you should be clear and confident about your choice of experiencing yoga.

And remember, please: there are many different kinds of yoga, and many different kinds of yoga instructors. Most of them are great; a handful of them may be well-intentioned, but may lack some of the foundation that they need in order to teach.

Remember always: no yoga instructor that you work with should ever humiliate you, degrade you, insult you, or make you feel inferior.

If you encounter the 1 in a 1000 who has not yet achieved the personal development that he/she needs in order to effectively teach, then remember: there are always other teachers!

The goal here is to make you happy, healthy, and confident. These criteria should be a part of all of your yoga experiences from day one.

Consistency

For you to enjoy every benefit of your commitment to practicing yoga, please note that consistency and regularity are the keys. You can't go into one session and skip three or four just because you're sore, had an unexpected engagement, or were too stressed out.

For the body and mind to change, you need to practice yoga consistently. Remove all obstacles, real or imagined and stay committed. Your rewards will be better health, better emotional balance, and a happier, more fulfilled life!

CHAPTER 4- YOGA POSES FOR BEGINNERS

Yoga positions for beginners are quite easy to learn. If you have not experienced any yoga session or have not seen one, which is not a problem.

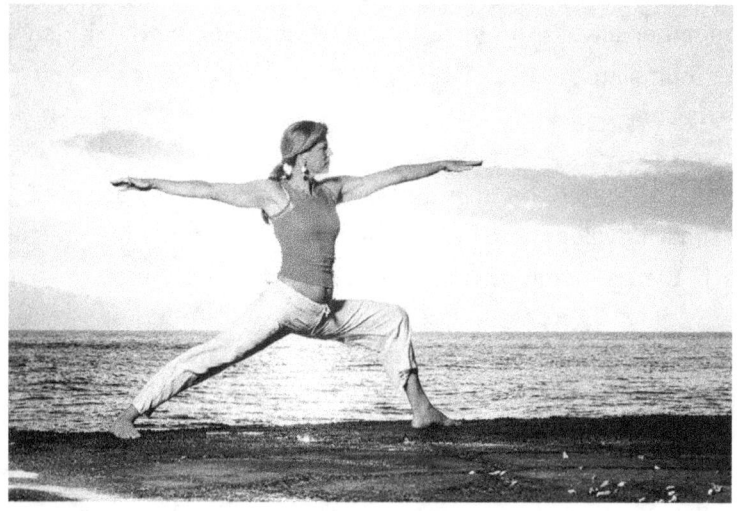

Practitioners have talked about the unification of the mind, body and spirit. They claimed that this will be acquired through the practice of yoga exercises and techniques.

If it is your first time to hear about yoga, you will of course wonder how these exercises are done and how it looks like. Since you are a beginner, you will also definitely ask what kind of positions will be best for you.

Yogis have believed that the mind and the body are bonded into a unified structure. This belief has never failed and changed through time. Yoga has extensively performed an amazing procedure of

Rajesh Vishwani

healing oneself through harmony. This can be successfully done if you are in a proper environment.

With the great effects of yoga, the doctors have been convinced that yoga has some therapeutic results and can be recommended for people who have illnesses that are hard to cure.

If you have some illness that has been with you for a long time, you can practice the yoga positions for beginners and apply it to yourself.

If you want to practice the yoga positions for beginners, you must believe that yoga is effective and will help you to be cured or be refreshed.

Yoga is not just a recent application. It has been practiced and applied a long time ago and up to the present, the people are benefiting a lot from it.

Investigations and researches have been implemented to prove that yoga can be helpful in the healing process.

Therefore, it has been proved that the yoga positions for beginners are extremely effective and useful when it comes to maintaining a high level of joint flexibility. Although the yoga positions for beginners are just simple and basic, it can slowly bring up a healthy lifestyle and bring more when it is practiced over and over again.

The yoga positions for beginners are very interesting and exciting to perform. Beginners will never find it hard to keep up with the exercises because it is just simple. The technique of yoga gives a very big contributing factor to our internal glands and organs. It also includes the parts of the human body which are barely stimulated.

Yoga For Beginners

If you want to learn the yoga positions for beginners, you can learn it easily at home or at school where yoga is taught.

Some basic yoga positions for beginners include standing poses, seated poses, forward and backward bends, balance and twisting. These yoga positions for beginners are not that far from those who are used to practicing yoga. Only that the extreme poses and positions are handled at the latter part of the exercise.

The time duration in executing the positions is also lessened because a beginner cannot fully cope up with a longer time exposure in practice. Rest is required of the beginner, so that he will not be drained easily to prepare the body for further positions.

Since you are a beginner, the most important thing you should understand is self discipline. Yoga is not just doing yoga and executing the poses. If you haven't mastered the basics yet, do not jump into the complex stages and positions because you will not feel the essence of executing the yoga positions for beginners.

Handling the Various Yoga Positions

There are a lot of yoga positions and poses that is built to improve posture.

Yoga positions have a lot of benefits such that it aims to improve our posture and give us a straight figure.

Sometimes, we might not notice ourselves in a crooked figure. If we practice that for a long time and not do anything about it, expect to have a crooked bone in the future.

Yoga positions are good to strengthen our body, giving focus to the thighs, knees and the ankles. If you get used to practicing yoga positions every day, it is expected that your bones respond immediately.

The abdomen and the buttocks are considered a major turn on for both genders. For the male, it is ideal to keep up a good abdomen of the abs. This makes it more appealing to the women.

Having a good butt matters to some women too, a lot of them are practicing in order to gain a lot of figure and shape in their body.

Yoga positions amazingly relieve sciatica. These are some pain that cannot be prevented. If you do yoga once in a while and even regularly, perhaps you will not feel any back or muscle pain.

Here are some techniques on how to maintain a good yoga position. Just follow these steps in order for you to fully understand yoga positions and be able to execute it in the proper manner.

1. You should stand with the bases of your big toes touching and the heels should be slightly apart. You must lift and spread your toes slowly and the balls of your feet too. Then after, you need to lay them softly down on the floor. Rock yourself back and forth and even side to side. You may gradually reduce this swaying to maintain a standstill, with your weight balanced evenly on your feet.

2. Hardening your thigh muscles and then lifting the knee caps is next. Do it without hardening your lower belly. Lift the inner ankles to make stronger the internal arches, then picture a line of energy all the way up along your inner thighs up to your groins. From there through the core of your neck, torso, and head, and out through the crown of your head. You should turn the upper thighs slowly inward.

Make your tailbone longer toward the floor and raise the pubis in the direction of the navel.

3. Push your shoulder blades into your back, then broaden them crossways and discharge them down your back. Without roughly pushing your lower front ribs forward, lift the top of your sternum straight toward the ceiling. Broaden your collarbones. Suspend your arms alongside the torso.

4. You should balance the crown of your head unswervingly over the middle of your pelvis, with the base of your chin analogous to the floor, throat soft, and the tongue broad and plane on the floor of your mouth. Make your eyes look softer.

5. Tadasana is usually the initial yoga position for all the standing poses. Applying Tansana is useful, especially in applying the poses. Staying in the pose for 30 seconds up to 1 minute, then breathing easily keeps it satisfactory.

Just follow these simple figures and you are sure that you are doing the right yoga positions.

There are a lot of yoga poses and you might wonder if some are still exercised and applied. The answer is yes. Yoga poses function and perform differently. Each pose is designed to develop one's flexibility and strength.

Here are some of the yoga poses that are commonly used:

Standing Poses

Standing is one of the important yoga poses. This type of pose is helpful in aligning your body and your feet. This is also very useful in improving and maintaining a good posture. It is an advantage because if you have a bad posture, your backbones can be stretched and straightened without noticing it. Standing poses help in giving strength to your legs and at the same time increase elasticity in your legs and hips because they are all connected to each other.

Seated Poses

These types of yoga poses increase your lower back and hip's flexibility. This also strengthens your back. This adds suppleness to your knees, groin, ankle and most especially your spine. Another advantage is that it helps you to breathe in deep which gives you that calm and peaceful feeling.

Forward Bends

This type helps you in stretching the hamstrings and your lower back also strengthening it. This lessens the tension found in your neck, shoulder, back and increase flexibility in your spine. Calmness is also achieved in this type of pose.

Back bends are amazingly helpful in opening your chest, hips and even the rib cage. This is helpful in strengthening and making your arms shoulders stronger. At the same time, it simultaneously increases your flexibility and elasticity in your shoulders. The great thing is that it helps to relieve the tension from the front of your body up to your hips and it increases your spinal ability. Your spinal cord is one thing that is important in your body so you need to take good care of it.

Back Bends

Notice that the forward bends are challenging because the exercise gives you a nice feeling and it can cause to fix some injuries. In this type of position, you can use a prop like the strap or the black because it will be very helpful.

Balance

Balance poses are very challenging. People who do yoga get too excited in performing balances. This is good because the fun that the person acquires helps him to live up his spirit and enlighten his soul. Balance is helpful in improving your posture. In improving your posture, the spinal cord is elongated which helps to keep yourself from some injuries and falling over.

Balance helps in training your ability to focus on your main goal and attention. However, attention should be obtained at the ultimate level because if your concentration is weak, for sure you cannot perform this type of pose.

Balance is one of the yoga poses that people truly appreciate and exert effort to. Along with the balance poses comes the twist which extremely releases tension all over your body. The tension in your spine is made clear. Twisting may seem to be hard to obtain. It is important to execute twists on both sides of the body so that the balance and alignment is obtained.

Taking note of these yoga poses will help you get along with yoga perfectly. Keep in mind that concentration is your main key if you want to be successful in doing these yoga poses.

CHAPTER 5- ACCESSORIES & EQUIPMENT USED FOR YOGA

The popularity of yoga has given rise to an industry that specializes in yoga equipment, accessories and clothes. The internet is a true marketplace of things yoga and product lines are as varied and diverse as the many teachings and postures of yoga.

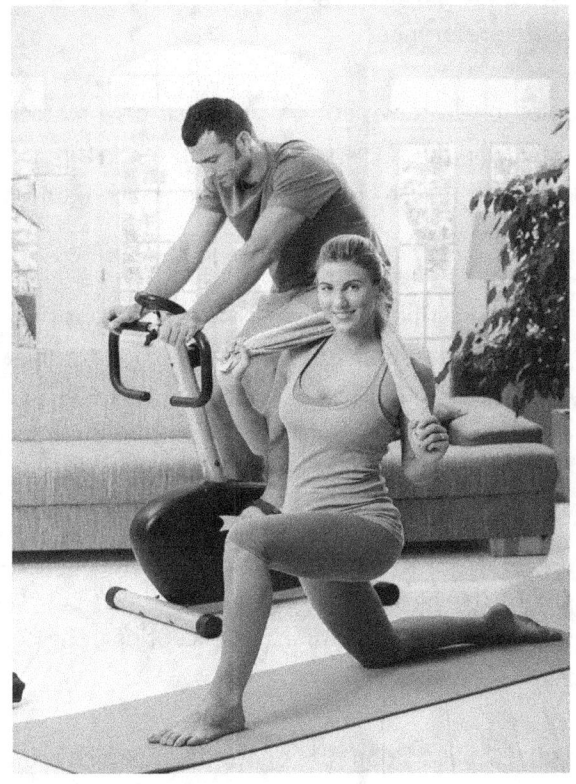

If you've ventured into your neighborhood sporting goods store, or even a department store, you've likely seen an array of yoga equipment that features very happy and peaceful looking people sitting on a yoga mat, or using a yoga towel. Indeed, for someone interested in yoga, this is like a kid in a candy store. There has never been a time in the marketplace where yoga equipment was so easy to find, and indeed, so affordable!

With that being said, it can be rather confusing as to which equipment does what. They all seem to have such happy looking people in the packaging; how do you know what's worth investing your money on?

Well, ultimately, the answer to that important question will be determined by the kind of yoga that you want to experience, and also, your own preferences.

Some people, for example, don't want to sit on a mat; they prefer the firmness of the floor. Other people find that sitting on the floor is painful and can lead to back and tailbone ache; and as such, a yoga mat is essential.

So, rather than prescribing here what you should buy and what you shouldn't, let's instead focus on the various neat things that you can easily buy, and you can use this information to help you make a wise decision.

Yoga Mats

Let's start with the famous yoga mat. Now, as a general rule (to which there will always, of course, be exceptions): be careful with the supermarket version.

A good yoga mat has a good grip on the floor, which is important if you have to perform complicated maneuvers and postures. They typically measure about 2 feet in width, and are available in a slew of rainbow colors.

There are yoga mats to fit all levels from beginner to advanced, and you have a choice of thickness. Many yoga stores will provide mats with efficient cushioning. Yoga mats are also available for children.

Yoga Towel

Don't forget your yoga towel. There are also skidless towels and some manufacturers make super absorbent ones – also, in what some retailers call, "chakra colors."

Yoga Bags

Yoga bags look rectangular – almost tubular – they are designed to hold your yoga mat and towel and other accessories.

Most products have a shoulder strap and are made of different materials, nylon being a common one. There are low end yoga bags retailing for $12.00 and they go up to $50.00, depending on make and size.

Yoga Straps

Those who do a lot of yoga flexibility routines often opting for yoga straps. These straps help them stretch their limbs, and to hold poses longer.

Yoga Sandbags and Bolsters

There are also yoga sandbags and bolsters that help your body balance and provide support as you perform your poses, stretches and positions. They are also available in many colors.

Yoga Medication Cushions, Chairs, Benches, and Pillows

The website www.yoga.com sells kits that include what they call "cosmic meditation cushion", which is advertised as ideal for peaceful medication. There's the back jack meditation chair (no legs) with firm upright back for support. There are also meditation benches (in different shapes) and the breathing (prayanama) pillow.

Yoga Balls

Balls are good for building strength, achieve balance and tone muscles. These fun yoga balls sell for about $25.00, and many dancers and physical therapists use yoga balls for a variety of movements, including: backbends, restorative poses and hip openers. Many balls can hold up to 600 pounds of weight.

And... remember: don't forget your air pump!

Yoga Blocks

These devices look like blocks, and have a mattress-feel to them. They're great for body movement extensions.

Yoga Videos/DVDs

If you're pressed for time, feel a bit shy about attending a public yoga class, or just want to have an idea of how yoga is practiced, yoga videos/DVDs are a great way to get initiated into yoga.

A great advantage of yoga videos is you can watch the clips over and over again until you've mastered the techniques correctly.

Rajesh Vishwani
Yoga Music

Consider trying yoga music to help you meditate better, breathe deeper, and hold those positions longer.

To name a few titles: Slow Music for Yoga, Tibetan Sacred Temple Music, Shiva Station, Nectar, Fragrance of the East, etc.

There is also yoga music for trance dance and yoga flow, chants and mantras and audio books.

Yoga Clothing

Though not mandatory for class, many yoga participants want an all-yoga attire to complement their yoga practice. Most beginners, however, come in a loose-fitting cotton T-shirt and comfortable leggings.

In choosing the perfect yoga clothes, of course they should be comfortable and made to give you a relaxing effect.

The best yoga clothes are those that allow you to freely move and prevent instances of distraction and disturbance when you are having your practice. They need to feel good on your skin so that you will be free from irritations.

Yoga clothes are an important accessory because it sets you into the mood. If you don't have the perfect set of yoga clothes, your day of practicing will be not be good.

During a heavy practice, it is expected that you will sweat too much. Some people don't really sweat too hard, but if you do, you should wear absorbent clothes so that the sweat on your body will be minimized and give you a dry feeling.

When you are all covered by sweat, you will have that sticky feel which keeps you uncomfortable and sometimes feel scratchy.

Although yoga clothes don't need to look that good, it is still important that you wear attractive ones so that you will have a good look and feel. Confidence is also an affecting factor in practicing. If you wear good yoga clothes, then you will not feel discriminated. So choose the best clothes that will match with your personality.

In practicing yoga, there is no requirement in choosing your clothes. If you want to show off some skin, it's up to you. If you have a body with good shape, you can wear fitting shirts and pants.

If you don't have that figure, but think that you have the guts, no one will scold you. After all, you're the one who carries your body as long as you can handle it.

Here are the common things you need when looking for in yoga clothing:

1. **Yoga Tops** – first thing you should consider in choosing a yoga top is that it should not fall on your face. Tops are designed to let you move freely and not be distracted when doing the exercise. If you are going to wear tee shirts, it should not be that long and should not cover the lower part of your body. This is important in checking the alignment of your lower body because you can see whether your knees and ankles are aligned properly. Most women wear sports bras so that in doing some movements, they are sure that it holds them securely and prevent chances of falling out when stretching.

2. **Yoga Pants** – Choosing your yoga pants is quite delicate. The texture and surface of some pants may not give you a

comfortable feel. The length of the pants is one of the things to consider in choosing it. Some pants are long that it reaches your ankles. If this is not comfortable to you, you should wear pants that are below your knees. This allows you to move freely.

3. **Yoga Shorts** – this is a good choice if you are practicing hot yoga or known as the Bikram Yoga. This type of yoga is done in a room at a high temperature. Wearing shorts will let go of the heat inside your body.

Choosing your yoga clothes doesn't mean that it has to be expensive. What is important is that you feel good and comfortable deep inside.

CHAPTER 6- CONCLUSION

The journey of yoga is one that is always an introduction; and hence, the title of this book is a little bit of a pleasant, Zen-like joke. There is no end to yoga; it is a constant process of discovering yourself, and energizing your body to give it optimal health.

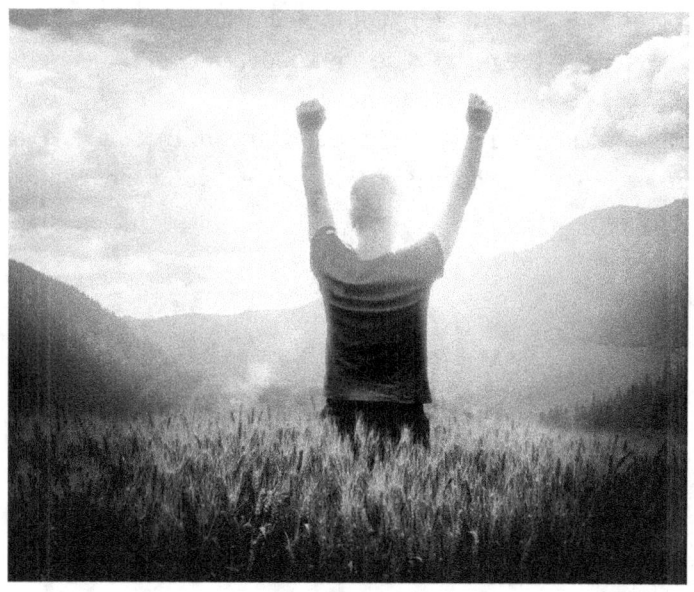

With that being said, for purely practical purposes, it's just fine to refer to something as an introduction to yoga, and hopefully this book has been a pleasant eye-opener for you.

Among other things, this book ideally:

Clarified for you that yoga is not a religion and therefore does not request or require you to change your faith.

Helped you understand the benefits of yoga; benefits that range from physical, to emotional, to psychological improvements.

Rajesh Vishwani
Helped you understand that yoga is not an "overnight thing", but takes consistency, commitment, and routine in order to deliver all of the benefits that you deserve

Helped you understand the various different kinds of yoga available to you (and all of these forms are available in the west, though some of the less popular one might only be centered in large urban areas).

Provided you with an overview of the various equipment that you can purchase (if you wish!) to enhance and improve your yoga journey.

In closing – we won't say concluding, since there's no end to this journey! – Let's enjoy the sage words of Swami Akhilananda, who very poetically describes the power and joy that people who attentively follow a yogi path experience.

(Please note, too, that if you don't like the usage of the word God in the quote below, simply replace it with something that fits within your own preference; the meaning and intent will remain the same).

"The real mystic who has spiritual realizations or super conscious experiences becomes extremely interested in his fellow beings as he finds the expression of God in them.

A mystic feels the presence of God everywhere and so he takes a loving interest not only in human beings but also in other beings."

ABOUT THE AUTHOR

Rajesh Vishwani lives yoga. He practices every morning and evening. He never used to be like this and used to be one of those individuals that were on the fast path to destroying himself. He used to party every night and had no concern about his future.

After his father became deathly ill, he came to the realization that life was much more than what he was making of it. He then started to find a way to normalize his life. That is how he found yoga. It was calming and peaceful and he felt so much better at the end of the day. He shares his own transformation that he experienced through yoga through his books.

www.ingramcontent.com/pod-product-compliance
Lightning Source LLC
Chambersburg PA
CBHW071133280526
45787CB00003B/1271